VIROLOGY
STUDY GUIDE

CONTENTS

INTRODUCTION

It's almost exam time and you are in panic mode!
Relax!
It's not the end of the world yet, but it might be if you
FAIL this course!
KIDDING!
Stay calm, just breathe, it's not as bad as you think. Take it one page at a time.

This book will provide you with some useful tricks and summaries.

Good Luck!

P.s If you are trying to learn everything one week before the exam let's just say you might have to ....(insert emoji)! Just kidding! Just maximize your study time and learn what's relevant.

Please be aware that this book aids you in condensing and understanding the material however it is UP TO YOU to find the correct answers to the QUESTION sections as you read through the material here, online, from a textbook or from lectures you attend. Being active in answering these questions will assist you in gaining and maintaining the basic knowledge of Virology. GOODLUCK

WHAT IS A VIRUS?

A **virus** is an acellular organism with genetic material protected by a protein shell that infects living host cells. The word virus was derived from a Greek word that means 'poison.'

WHAT PROPERTIES DO VIRUSES HAVE?
- No enzymes
- No protein synthesis machinery
- Cannot make ATP
- Single nucleic acid type, RNA/DNA
- Needs host cell's metabolic machinery
- Metabolically inert
- Not considered to be alive

Remember: You need living cells so that the virus can grow. Viruses cannot be grown on sterile media but require presence of specific host cells.

WHICH VIRUS WAS FIRST DESCRIBED?
In 1898 Foot and Mouth disease was described. The virus that causes this disease is in the family known as *Picornaviridae*.

What other viruses may have been described or discovered around this time?

TASK:- Consider Yellow Fever virus , Rous Sarcoma virus, Polio virus and the virus that causes Chicken pox. When do you think these viruses were described or discovered?

VIRUS CLASSIFICATION

ORDER

VIRIDAE

FAMILY

VIRINAE

SUBFAMILY

VIRUS

GENUS

SPECIES

STRAIN TYPE

*Note that ORDER, FAMILY, GENUS written in italics

WHICH VIRUS FAMILIES HAVE SUBFAMILIES?

Poxviridae
Parvoviridae
Paramyxoviridae
Herpesviridae
Reoviridae
Retroviridae

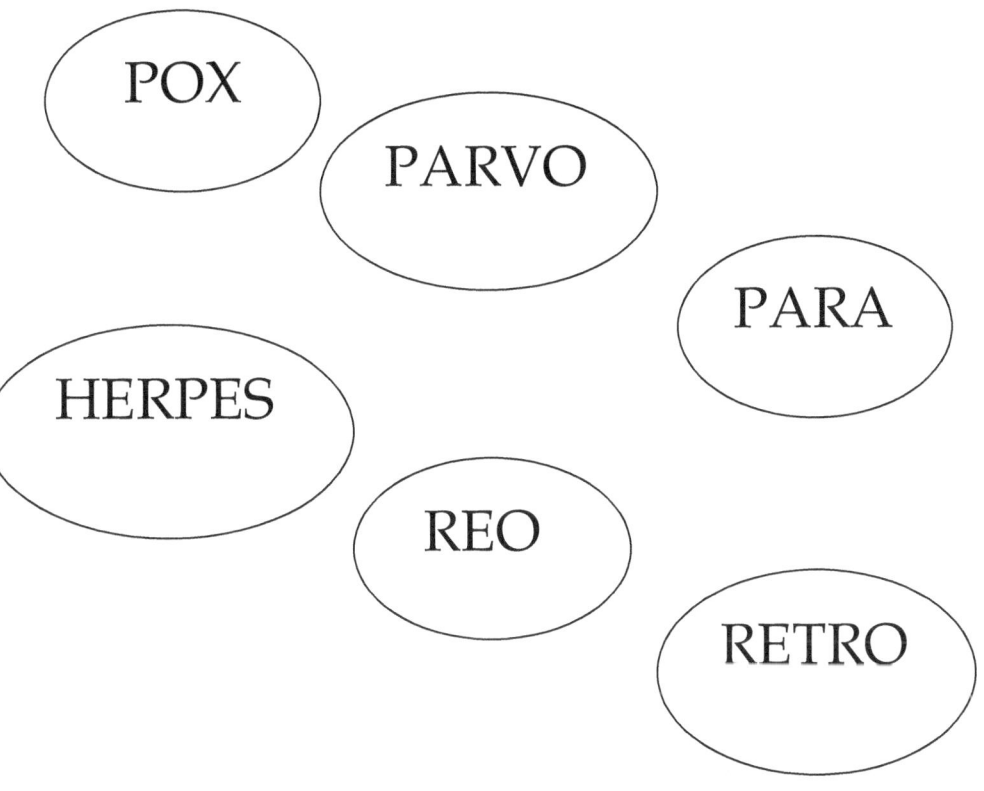

DNA VIRUS FAMILIES

ds DNA

PHAP

pox, herpes, adeno,papova - VIRIDAE

ss DNA

PARVO

Partial ds DNA

HEPADNA

DNA VIRUSES

PLUS SENSE RNA VIRUS FAMILIES

CTF Pi Ca

Corona, Toga, Flavi, Picorna, Calici – VIRIDAE

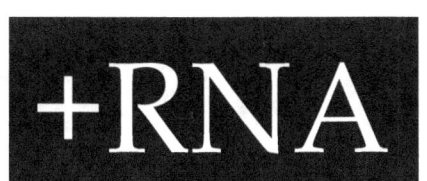

Single Stranded Plus sense RNA

RETRO

Diploid +RNA

Diploid plus sense RNA

MINUS SENSE RNA VIRUS FAMILIES

PRF

Paramyxo, Rhabdo, Filo– VIRIDAE

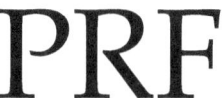

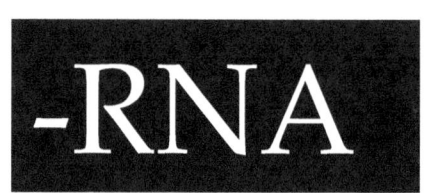 Non-segmented

Single stranded Minus sense RNA

BOAReo

Bunya, Orthomyxo, Arena, Reo– VIRIDAE

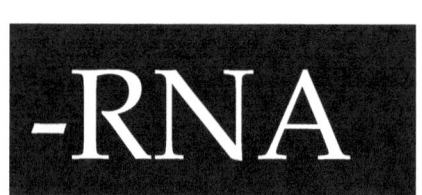 Segmented

Minus sense RNA

PRF are part of The **ORDER** called *MONONEGAVIRALES*

SEGMENTED MINUS SENSE RNA VIRUSES

SEGMENTED virus means a virus that has two or more pieces of nucleic acid packaged in the same particle

BOAReo

FAMILY	BUNYA	ORTHOMYX	ARENA	REO
Genome	+ss or -ss	-ss	+ss or (+/-)ss	ds
Capsid	Helical	Helical	Helical	Icosahedral
Envelope	Yes	Yes	Yes	No
Segments	3	8	2	12
VIRUS (Genus)	Hantavirus Phlebovirus	Influenzavirus A Influenzavirus B Influenzavirus C	Arenavirus *LCM-LASV-Complex *Tacaribe Complex	Rotavirus
Species	Hantaan virus Puumala virus Sin Nombre virus Rift Valley fever virus	Influenza virus A Influenza virus B Influenza virus C	Lassa fever virus LCMV Muchupo virus	RotavirusA RotavirusB RotavirusC

**Underlined viruses represent the TYPE SPECIES of their Genus

POSITIVE, NEGATIVE, DNA, RNA

Positive sense means that the nucleotide sequence is the same as mRNA.
Task: Can you name some positive sense viruses.

....
....
....
....

Negative sense means that the nucleotide is not the same as the mRNA.
Task: Can you name some negative sense viruses.

....
....
....
....

Ambisense means that there is a mixture of the two. Therefore 5′ ends are positive and the 3′ ends are negative.
Task: Can you name DNA virus that does not replicate in the nucleus?

....
....
....
....

DNA genomes are usually large and usually replicate in the nucleus.
Task: Can you name DNA virus that does not replicate in the nucleus?..
....

RNA genomes are usually small and usually replicate in the cytoplasm.

Task: Can you name DNA virus that does not replicate in the nucleus?...
....
... ...

Viral Tropism is the ability of a virus to infect specific populations of cells within an organ.

Task: Can you name some viruses and which populations of cells they preferentially infect.

... ...
... ...
... ...
... ...
... ...
... ...
... ...
... ...
... ...
... ...
... ...
... ...
... ...
... ...
... ...
... ...
... ...
... ...

Hint:- Consider Rabies virus, Human Immunodeficiency virus, Hepatitis B virus, Rotavirus A, Ebola virus, West Nile virus, Herpes Simplex virus, Dengue virus, smallpox virus (Variola)

QUESTIONS

1) Which virus families belong to the order Mononegavirales? Give examples of their virus species.
2) Name the Type species for Hantavirus?
3) Which other Species is found in the Genus Hantavirus?
4) Name the type species for Influenzavirus A?
5) Name three things that make Reoviridae family different from the other segmented minus sense?
6) Is Rift Valley fever virus the Type Species for the Genus Phlebovirus?
7) Which virus family has the least segments?
8) Which virus families have subfamilies?
9) List at least three plus sense virus species?
10) Which Arenavirus is distributed worldwide?
11) Which Arenavirus is distributed in West Africa?
12) Name one virus family that is ambisense, name its type genus. Lastly, Name its type species if it has one?
13) What does 'ambisense' mean?
14) Influenza A virus is proposed to have how many segments?
15) Which virus causes mild respiratory infections - Influenza A or Influenza C?
16) How are Bunyaviruses transmitted?
17) In relation to Influenza describe antigenic drift and antigenic shift. Which one is responsible for pandemics?
18) Which virus families have a vaccine?
19) What's the main difference between RNA & DNA polymerase
20) Give examples of virus species that require a vector for transmission.

HINT:- Be careful when answering questions. If you are asked to name a virus species and you name a virus family- **THIS IS WRONG!** Check that you have answered questions carefully and that you are clear of the differences between ORDER, FAMILY, GENUS etc.

TASK:- Consider visiting the world health organization (WHO) website and browse through their current information on these viruses. Virology is a field that can drastically change year to year (example. Classifications) - therefore it is important that you stay up to date with the information concerning these viruses. Make notes of the most important aspects of each virus or virus family!

VIRAL REPLICATION

1. Attachment
2. Penetration
3. Uncoating of nucleic acid
4. Early viral protein expression
5. Replication of viral genome
6. Expression of late viral proteins
7. Assembly of genome and virion
8. Egress
9. Release

Task: Take a very close look at the replication cycles of viruses that are of interest to you. Do they follow the pattern above? What is unique to Herpesviridae, Retroviridae (HIV) and Hepatitis B virus?

....
....
....
....
....
....
....
....
....

Is there a link between the egress mechanism to the absence or presence of an envelope? (Budding versus Lysis)

....
....
....
....

TRANSMISSION

FOMITE – ANY OBJECT OR SUBSTANCE CAPABLE OF CARRYING INFECTIOUS ORGANISMS AND HENCE TRANSFERRING THEM FROM ONE INDIVIDUAL TO ANOTHER

Which viruses can be spread by fomites?

....
....
....
....
....
....
....

Virus transmission is split into three types

1) **Horizontal** – Host to Host / Fomites / Animal bites/ Body fluids

2) **Vertical** – Mother to Child – BreastMilk/During Birth / Through the placenta

3) **Vector** – Host to animal to host
   Can you give examples of what type of animals? Which animals or insects are involved as vectors in which disease transmission?

   ....
   ....

   Hint: Bunyavirus, Dengue virus , Arboviral diseases, rodents, monkeys, monkeypox virus

4) Have monkeys given humans any diseases? Which?

   ....

TRANSMISSION, MODE, VIRUS

Type of transmission	Mode of transmission	Virus
Horizontal	Animal bites	Rabies
Horizontal	Skin	HSV
Horizontal	Blood	HIV
Horizontal	Urine	Hantavirus
Horizontal	Saliva	Influenza A
Horizontal	Fecal Matter	HAV
Horizontal	Tears	Ebola virus
Horizontal	Mucosal surfaces	HSV
Vertical	Birthcanal	HIV

Task:- Add to the table! Considering the following words
- Transplacental – What type of transmission, Which virus
- Breast milk - What type of transmission, Which virus
- Poliovirus – What type of transmission and what mode
- Epstein Barr virus- What type of transmission and what mode
- Hepatitis B virus- What type of transmission and what mode
- Hepatitis A virus - What type of transmission and what mode
- Rotavirus - What type of transmission and what mode
- Yellow fever virus - What type of transmission and what mode

Keep in mind that the **portals of viral entry** include
Eyes
Mouth – Respiratory tract and Alimentary canal
Skin
Urogenital tract
Anus

Questions –Why is the skin an effective barrier against viruses?..
....

Can Rabies be transmitted from an organ transplant? Has there been any reports of this? Can Zika be transmitted through sexual intercourse? (Be careful here! Check latest data)
....
....

We know that viruses thrive in damp areas, which areas of the human body are damp enough to allow viruses to proliferate. **Does the human body have any mechanism to prevent this from happening?**
....
....
....
....
....
Hint: Think of areas like the genital tract and alimentary canal?

The fact that humans are exposed to a vast amount of viruses and bacteria daily but hardly become ill everyday suggests that there are barriers or mechanisms implemented to protect the body.
Can you list some of these mechanisms?
....
....
....
....
Hint: Think of the Eye, Respiratory tract, Enzymes, Temperature, pH, sinuses

ONCE THE VIRUS CROSSES BARRIERS THEN WHAT?

Viremia – when the virus enters the body and spreads throughout the host's body via blood. It is simply defined as the presence of viruses in the blood.

Viremia usually follows primary replication which occurs at the initial site of infection. Viruses can spread through the host via the **bloodstream** or the **nervous system.** Which viruses can spread through the bloodstream or nervous system?

Bloodstream

....
....
....

Nervous system

....
....
....

Hint: Think of viruses that cross
Epithelial barrier
Blood to tissue/brain barrier

Which viruses can you detect or diagnose from blood?...
....
....
....
....

Which viruses show cytopathic effect?

....
....

CPE – structural changes in host cells caused by viral invasion. Cell death, cell fusion, multinucleation or growth.

MAGNIFYING GLASS ON EACH VIRUS

For the viruses you wish to study it is important to have a general idea of their taxonomy, classification, components of its virion including genome composition. In addition it is important to know the replication strategy, transmission, epidemiology, diagnosis and treatment. Essentially virology requires you to master the most important details of each viruses specially those details that are highly unique to that virus. It may seem overwhelming at first but it can be done. One virus at a time!

This book will not discuss each virus in detail however we will provide some questions that may assist you in determining whether you have grasped the basic knowledge of some of the viruses. In addition we will share some interesting facts or summaries that are unique to certain viruses or virus families.

BIOWEAPON VIRUSES

Poxviridae, viruses causing encephalitis and viruses causing haemorrhagic fever are included in the list of viruses that can be used in biowarfare. This is probably because they share properties such as high lethality, highly contagious, predictable incubation periods with symptoms that appear as symptoms of other common but non harmful or minor diseases. The most important factor is that humans are the only reservoir.

Task:-

Name two Genuses under Poxviridae as well as their respective type species?

Which Type species is used in the pox vaccinations

....

....

....

....

List virus families that fall under viruses that cause haemorrhagic fever (5Families known)

List virus families that fall under viruses that cause encephalitis...

....

....

POX VIRUS

Pox virus has more than one membrane and known to be brick shaped. **It also replicates in the cytoplasm**. Why is this so surprising given what you know about the nucleic acid of Poxviridae?

…………………………………………………………………………

…………………………………………………………………………

…………………………………………………………………………

Variolation – The use of ground powdered smallpox scabs to inoculate patients and immunize them against smallpox (Variola). Practice which was first used by the Chinese.

E.Jenner then scientifically proved that infection with cowpox protected against smallpox. Why would this be possible?...

....

....

Hint: Take a look at the classification of Variola (Smallpox) and Cowpox

Luckily variolation was soon replaced with live vaccines and WHO announced the eradication in **1980.** (Visit the WHO page and take a look at the vaccination schedules for smallpox the schedules have been worldwide).

Smallpox looks like other diseases such as Varicella and Herpes Zoster.

By looking at a patient how can you differentiate between smallpox and chickenpox?

…………………………………………………………………………

…………………………………………………………………………

…………………………………………………………………………

…………………………………………………………………………

Which virus family do we find Varicella (Chickenpox)?

....

....

Which viral infections would lead you to be under quarantine? How long is the period of quarantine?

………………………………………………………………………

………………………………………………………………………

………………………………………………………………………

………………………………………………………………………

………………………………………………………………………

Quarantine – enforced isolation of an infected person or person exposed to a communicable disease.

Pandemic – An epidemic that affects multiple geographic areas at the same time worldwide.

Epidemic – A widespread outbreak of an infectious disease where many people are infected at the same time.

What are the contributing factors that predispose a virus to become an epidemic? Or pandemic?

………………………………………………………………………

………………………………………………………………………

………………………………………………………………………

………………………………………………………………………

………………………………………………………………………

………………………………………………………………………

………………………………………………………………………

………………………………………………………………………

………………………………………………………………………

Explain how Influenza becomes epidemic or pandemic?

………………………………………………………………………

………………………………………………………………………

………………………………………………………………………

………………………………………………………………………

How are the vaccines for Influenza made? (Check the WHO website for the latest vaccinations for Influenza and take a note of their contents i.e standard nomenclature)

………………………………………………………………………
………………………………………………………………………
………………………………………………………………………
………………………………………………………………………
………………………………………………………………………

Hint: Standard nomenclature system

Type, host of origin, geographical origin, strain number and year of isolation, serotypes of HA and NA is given parenthetically.

Which other viruses despite Influenza result in respiratory tract infections? State virus family and species (or type species)

………………………………………………………………………
………………………………………………………………………
………………………………………………………………………
………………………………………………………………………
………………………………………………………………………
………………………………………………………………………

Hint: Some are in the genus Herpesvirus, Picornavirus, Paramyxovirus

BALTIMORE

Task: Find out about this viral classification and fill in the grid above. Which Baltimore number are Retroviruses?

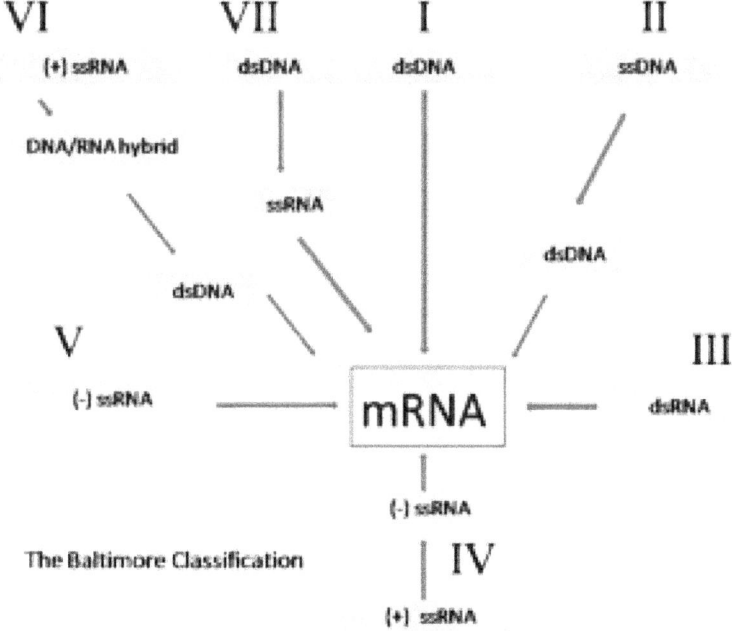

The Baltimore Classification

HEPATITIS ALPHABET

HEPATITIS VIRUS	BALTIMORE	VIRUS FAMILY	NUCLEIC ACID	SEVERITY
A	V	Picornaviridae	+ssRNA	Acute hepatitis
B	VII	Hepadnaviridae	dsDNA	Acute and Chronic
C	IV	Flaviviridae	+ssRNA	
D		Deltaviridae	-ssRNA	
E	IV	Hepeviridae	+ssRNA	Acute hepatitis
G	IV	Flavividae	+ssRNA	Infects humans but not known to cause disease

HEPATITIS VIRUS	TRANSMISSION	TRANSMISSION	VACCINATION
A	Enteral	Faecal-oral	Yes
B	Parenteral	Blood, Semen, Other body fluids	Yes
C	Parenteral	Blood	No
D	Parenteral	Co-infection with HBV	HBV-vaccine
E	Enteral	Contaminated water or food	China -yes
G		Blood, blood products, sexual and vertical transmission	No

HEPATITS ALPHABET

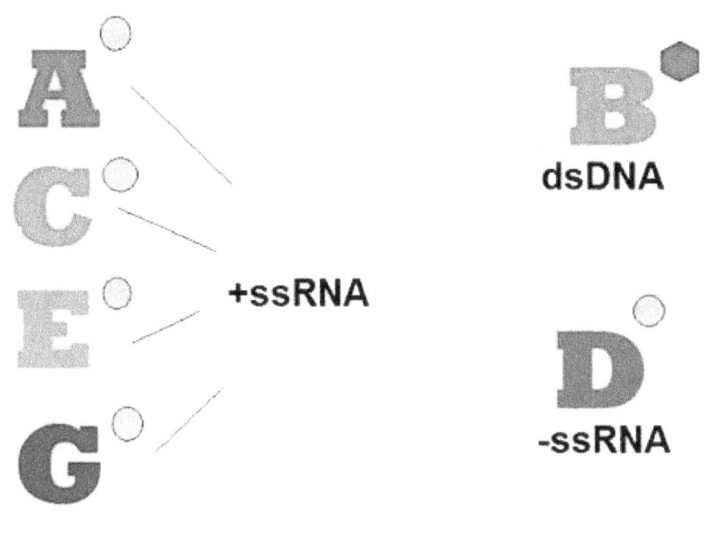

+ssRNA

dsDNA

-ssRNA

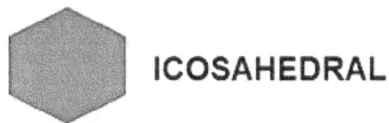 ICOSAHEDRAL

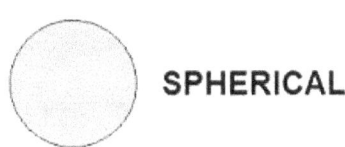 SPHERICAL

Task : - Which ones are enveloped or non-enveloped (naked).
Fil in this table below

A	
B	
C	
D	Enveloped
E	Non-enveloped
G	

Task : - Looking at the transmission pathways of Hepatitis viruses can you suggests methods of diagnosis, risk groups and preventative measures?

....

....

....

....

....

....

....

....

....

Is there one Hepatitis virus which is the most lethal? Which one and why?

....

....

....

Which hepatitis virus is more severe in pregnant women?

Yellow fever shares which virus family with which hepatitis virus?..

....

What do Polio virus and Hepatitis A virus have in common?

....

Aedes albopictus (Tiger mosquitoe) transmits which viruses (or diseases) that share the same virus family as one of the hepatitis viruses? Which hepatitis virus? The Tiger mosquito is also known to transmit chikungunya, from which virus family is chikungunya from and which other viruses do you know are in this family..

TONGUE TIED! RUBELLA, RUBIVIRUS, RUBEOLA, RUBULAVIRUS

Task: Simply define each of the words below. It may help you to differentiate the disease, genus, species etc…

Rubella
Rubivirus
Third disease / 3day measles
3 day Fever
Rubeola
Rubulavirus
Erythema Infectiosum
Roseolovirus
Roseola infantum
5th Disease
6th Disease
B19
Lassa fever virus
Lyssavirus

Which Genus do we find mumps and measles virus?
……………………………………………………………………
……………………………………………………………………
………………………………………………………………..........
Mumps virus shares a Genus with HPIV2,4 or HPIV1,3?
……………………………………………………………………
……………………………………………………………………

VIRUS FACTS

Make sure to check these facts with current data.

Flaviviridae and Arenaviridae lack poly-A tail

IRES found in Picornaviridae and Flaviviridae (HepC)

Ambisense virus families are Bunyaviridae and Arenaviridae

Filoviridae known to be the longest in size

Coronaviridae has the longest RNA genome

Poxvirus and Mimivirus are part of the largest viruses

Reoviridae has the most segments

Latency is seen in Adeno-associated viruses and Herpesviridae

Poxvirus is the most complex virus

Many viruses are treated with Ribavirin. Some of which include SARs-Cov, Lassa fever virus, Dengue fever virus

Bunyaviridae is known to not show cytopathic effects

Orthomyxoviridae is an RNA virus that replicates in the nucleus

Retroviruses have transcription in the nucleus and replicate in the cytoplasm

Bunyaviridae is the biggest member of viruses
Poxviridae are DNA viruses that have replication and transcription in the cytoplasm

Dengue fever virus and Enterovirus 71 both have biphasic fevers

Hepadnaviridae and Retroviridae both have reverse transcriptase

Circular genome is seen in hepadnaviridae (HepB), Herpesviridae (during latency) and Deltavirus (Hep D)

Virus family with packaging domain is Adenoviridae

Adenovirus has antitumour activity

Virus that intergrate into a specific location in human chromosome is AAV2

Viruses that you can catch by organ transplantation include HHV4, HHV5, Rabies virus, HGV and HCV

Task:- As you study your books and class material you will find more facts that you can add to the list

HERPESVIRIDAE
What's so special about the tegument in Herpesviridae?

....

		Subfamily & Genus
HHV-1	Herpes Simplex virus1	Alphaherpesvirinae Simplexvirus
HHV-2	Herpes Simplex virus2	Alphaherpesvirinae Simplexvirus
HHV-3	Varicella Zoster virus	Alphaherpesvirinae Varicellovirus
HHV-4	Epstein Barr virus	Gammaherpesvirinae Lymphocrytovirus
HHV-5	Human cytomegalovirus	Betaherpesvirinae Cytomegalovirus
HHV-6A, 6B, 7	Roseola infantum	Betaherpesvirinae Roseolovirus
HHV-8	Kaposi's sarcoma associated herpesvirus	Gammaherpesvirinae Rhadinovirus

Task:- How are each of these HHVs transmitted.

Hint: Place these options with a virus above. sexually, Body fluids, Contact with sores, blood, vertically at birth, saliva, organ transplant, vertical via germline, via birth by genitally infected mother, oral to oral, oral to genital, surfaces around mouth, blood transfusion, objects like toothbrush, contact from rash blisters

---

THE 6 SKIN RASH DISEASES

1) Measles
2) Scarlet fever
3) Rubella (3rd disease) (3day measles)
4) Filatov dukes disease
5) Erythema infectiosum (B19) (5th disease)
6) Roseola infantum (3day fever)

General Questions

1) How are adenoviruses and adeno-associated viruses different? Give examples of their virus species.

   ………………………………………………………………
   ………………………………………………………………
   ………………………………………………………………
   ………………………………………………………………
   ………………………………………………………………
   ………………………………………………………………

2) What is a naked virus? List 3 naked viruses? Are naked viruses sensitive to soap? Explain.

   ………………………………………………………………
   ………………………………………………………………
   ………………………………………………………………
   ………………………………………………………………
   ………………………………………………………………
   ………………………………………………………………

3) Budding can occur from which organelles or cell structures?

   ………………………………………………………………
   ………………………………………………………………
   ………………………………………………………………

4) B19 virus belongs to which family and what disease does it cause?

   ………………………………………………………………

5) Hantavirus or Hantaan virus is Genus or Type species. Which is which?

   ………………………………………………………………

6) What is the difference between Chronic and Latent?

7) Name two viruses that can be transferred from pigs to humans.

....

....

8) VSV is a good vector for Ebola vaccine. Why?

....

....

....

....

9) Rabies is what percent lethal? Is there a chance of survival once you catch the virus?

....

....

....

....

10) Which of the following have vaccine
    Yellow Fever
    Dengue Fever
    West Nile Fever
    Zika

11) Why does a dead vaccine not protect for long?

....

....

....

12) Which virus is older measles virus or HIV?............

13) Which virus is older Polio virus or smallpox virus?

....

14) Which virus was reported to be eradicated in 1980 by WHO?

....

....

15) What is an episomal virus?

....

....

16) What factors are required in order for a disease to be eradicated?

....

....

....

....

....

17) Why is there antibody enhancement with dengue and zika?

....

....

....

18) How does the poxvirus evade the immune system?

....

....

....

....

19) Why does having more segments make a virus more dangerous?

....

....

....

20) What is the difference between active and passive vaccine?

....

....

....

....

21) List four viruses with helical symmetry?

....

....

....

22) Define viroid and virosoide.

....
....
....
....
....

23) Since viruses cannot be propagated in cell culture what is used instead?

....
....
....

24) Which viral structures do Adenoviruses use to enter cells?

....

25) What are emerging viruses and how do they occur? Give examples.

....
....
....
....

26) Which clinical outcome is common in emerging viruses?

....
....

27) 25% of the common cold comes from which virus family?

....

28) What is the viral host of Lassa fever? ....

29) What is VSV-EBOV?

....
....
....
....

30) Give a brief description of Ebola virus pathology

....

31) Which virus family is bullet-shaped?

....

....

32) What are negri bodies and are related to which virus?

....

....

....

33) Which animals can spread a virus from the genus lyssavirus?

....

....

....

34) Name a virus family that is ssDNA? What is the type species and what disease/s does it cause?

....

....

35) Which is more contagious measles or chickenpox? What determines how contagious a virus is?

....

....

....

....

36) Which viruses are more likely to mutate RNA viruses or DNA viruses and why?

....

....

....

37) Does the same mosquitoe transmit West Nile fever and Dengue Fever?If not- which mosquitoes transmit these?

....

38) What is the significance of viral load during transmission?

....
....
....
....

39) Why is there no such thing as 100% vaccination of a population? Approximately what is average percentage that is vaccinated to eradicate a disease?

....
....
....
....

40) India has the highest prevalence of which virus. Rabies virus or Ebola virus?

....

41) What is a provirus?

....
....
....
....

42) Can HIV patients become resistant to their drugs? What is the solution?

....
....
....

43) Lentivirus vectors are used in gene therapy for which diseases? Give examples?

....

44) Draw the basic genomic structure of HIV?

45) Discuss which virus families or virus species are used in gene therapy and discuss their efficiency in gene therapy in terms of packaging capacity, transgene expression, interaction with host gene. What are the typical advantages and disadvantages for each?

Hint:- It may be easier to draw a table. Consider Retrovirus, Adenovirus, AAV, Parvoviridae, Herpesviruses

46) What is the Cre/loxP system

....
....
....

GENE TRANSFER VECTORS

	Adenovirus	Adeno-associated virus	Retrovirus
Efficient Gene Transfer	Yes	Yes	No
Host cell genome integration	No	No	Yes
Long term correction of chronic disorders	No	No	Yes
Therapeutic of high expression	Yes	Yes	No

Task:- Are there any other virus families that can be used in gene-therapy that are not in the table? What are their properties? Give an example of which species from which family is used and for therapy for which diseases?

END NOTE

It is important to understand that Virology is a large and although we have omitted some aspects we believe that active participation in the exercises in this book will give you a boost to an introduction in virology. We wish you a pleasant ride in your quest to conquer the world of viruses.

NOW GO STUDY!

GOOD LUCK

P.s As you study each virus topic in your curriculum Remember to always keep in mind the most important aspects of each virus. Also ask yourself questions as you go through the material this helps you process the logic behind each virus. It will also help you find links between some virus families or even interesting anomalies.

DON'T PANIC
JUST BREATHE
AND ALL THE BEST!

MY NOTES

....
....
....
....
....
....
....
....
....
....
....
....
....
....
....
....
....
....
....
....
....
....
....
....
....
....
....
....
....
....
....

www.ingramcontent.com/pod-product-compliance
Lightning Source LLC
Chambersburg PA
CBHW071241220526
45468CB00002B/954